A HOLISTIC APPROACH

TO CURING LYME DISEASE

Healing Lyme Disease Naturally

by

Dr. Earendil M. Spindelilus D.N.M., M.H., C.R., PSc.D

Table of Contents

LIST OF FIGURES

DEDICATION

To my wife and best friend Peggy, who has stood beside me and put up with all of my time spent getting one degree or certification after another.

I would also like to express my gratitude for all of the patients who have taught me so much about how to be a doctor.

Not all doctors are healers and not all healers are doctors.

CHAPTER 1

Introduction

The purpose of this book is to offer an alternative treatment for both acute and chronic Lyme disease. To date there are currently 300,000 new cases of Lyme reported in the United States each year. That is six times the reported new cases of HIV. It is the new pandemic of this century. Sadly, most doctors today are either not Lyme-literate or prefer to choose the conventional approach to treatment which is simply symptomatic with high doses of antibiotics. This method has been proven to offer no cure for this disorder and in the end bankrupts most patients. This book will explain in detail the etiology of Lyme current accepted conventional protocols, along with a treatment plan I have been using in practice for over 20 years. I will also be discussing successful case histories where patients were cured and remain so to this day.

For the past twenty years of practice, from top to bottom, I have treated everything from boo-boo toes to brain cancer. The past seven years we have run one of the largest Traditional Naturopathic medical centers in California called Tree Of Life Holistic Wellness Center. Using holistic, Naturopathic protocols we have seen amazing success in working with issues such as cancer, auto-immune including as M.S., Lupus, and such. But of all the disorders that have come through our door at the clinic, Lyme would rate as the most difficult and stubborn, and devastating I have witnessed. Another doctor I know of stated once that Lyme was more difficult to treat than cancer. There is some truth to that statement. The Borrelia bacteria, from my perspective, is the most evolved advanced I have come across. It has an amazing ability to trick the human immune system. If attacked, it will often change the outer protein shell to defeat the antibiotic or it may go into a "cyst" stage and "go to sleep" until the time when the body is weak and ready for another round of attacks.

For years I treated patients, often relying on their previous diagnosis. They would come in with "confirmed" diagnosis for Lupus, Multiple Sclerosis, Rheumatoid Arthritis, Fibromyalgia, Chronic Fatigue Syndrome, etc. I would begin a holistic set of treatments aimed at eliminating the disorders. While they would often find some improvement in their symptoms, the condition itself would persist, sometimes for months or years. Occasionally, they would appear cured, no longer symptomatic. They would leave the clinic happy and looking forward to a healthier life.

Sadly, within months they would return to the clinic as the "old" problem returned. This would often mystify me as I knew from past experience what I had prescribed would work every time for issues such as they presented. I knew in my heart that this should have worked, even in somewhat resistant patients, those who have issues following a protocol.

During this period of time I had begun studying and training in the protocols involving the diagnosis and treatment of Lyme Disease. I began to become suspicious that the original diagnosis from the previous doctors may not have been correct. I started asking patients if we could run a series of tests recommended by Dr. Burrascano, sometimes at a cost to the clinic. We were beginning to suspect there was more going on and when a patient could not afford it and had already spent a great deal of money within the medical system, we would cover the cost of the tests as we were not sure this was actually Lyme.

As it turned out, in so many of the cases, they had been misdiagnosed. It was not unusual for the patients to begin to cry, not from sorrow but joy at finally receiving an actual, correct diagnosis. I applied what I had learned about the manner with which this bacteria attacks the immune system, started treating the co-infections so often present, and we began to see positive, significant results.

Within this book, I will go over the protocols I have used over the years as well as actual case histories of just a few of our success stories. I will compare the success of conventional protocols versus those developed by the holistic community. There is indeed a place for both of us in the medical world as we each contribute to medical wisdom. This will also be the first book in a series detailing the natural, healing protocols for a wide variety of conditions, such as hypertension, diabetes, auto-immune and such. We hope you find this book helpful and please feel free to send me your success stories or personal observations you have experienced in coping with Lyme disease. The clinic's email is clinic@treeoflifehwc.com.

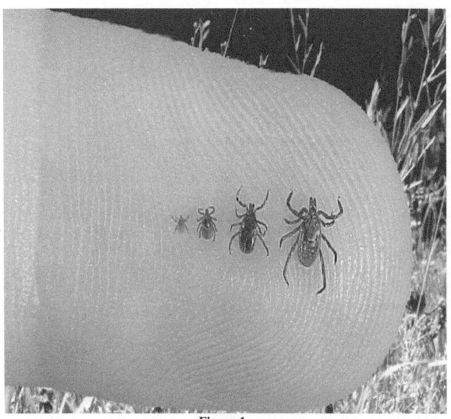

Figure 1

The stages of deer tick growth. Only stages 1 and 4 can transmit the bacteria.

1.1   What is Lyme Disease

In the 1960s and 1970s, something was very wrong in Connecticut. In a population of 12,000 living in three contiguous towns: Old Lyme, Lyme, and East Haddam, 39 children were diagnosed with juvenile rheumatoid arthritis and 12 adults were diagnosed with arthritis of unknown cause.
In 1975, frustrated by the lack of answers from their medical community, two mothers became patient advocates, gathering information from residents that they passed on to the Connecticut State Department of Health and the Yale School of Medicine.

In 1982, the agent responsible for Lyme disease was discovered by Willy Burgdorfer, who isolated spirochetes belonging to the genus Borrelia from the mid-guts of ticks infecting deer, other wild animals, and dogs.
Spirochetes are spiral-shaped bacteria that have been identified as early as 30,000 BC. The causative organism was named Borrelia burgdorferi (Bb), after its discoverer.

Following is a quote from JOSEPH J. BURRASCANO JR., M.D. as one of the best definitions for Lyme:

"I take a broad view of what Lyme Disease actually is. Traditionally, Lyme is defined an infectious illness caused by the spirochete, Borrelia burgdorferi (Bb). While this is certainly technically correct, clinically the illness often is much more than that, especially in the disseminated and chronic forms.

Instead, I think of Lyme as the illness that results from the bite of an infected tick. This includes infection not only with B. burgdorferi, but the many co-infections that may also result. Furthermore, in the chronic form of Lyme, other factors can take on an ever more significant role- immune dysfunction, opportunistic infections, coinfections, biological toxins, metabolic and hormonal imbalances, deconditioning, etc. I will refer to infection with B. burgdorferi as "Lyme Borreliosis" (LB), and use the designation "Lyme" and "Lyme Disease" to refer to the more broad definition I described above."

The vast majority of Lyme cases that I have treated over 19 years of practice fits well with the above definition. It is also correct to define it within the parameters of the secondary or co-infections. There have been cases when it was difficult to isolate the B. burgdorferi and yet the tests were clearly positive for such infections as the Babesia bacteria, a common secondary infection associated with Lyme.

Lyme on the march

Cases of Lyme disease have spread across the US as warmer winters encourage the ticks that carry it to move into new areas

2001   2005   2010   2015

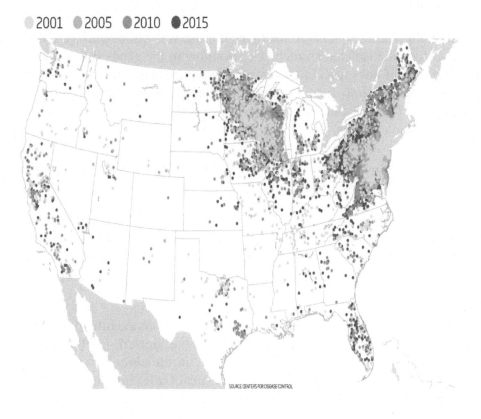

Figure 2.

1.2   Common Symptoms

Unfortunately, this disease is one of the great mimickers as it can appear as dozens of others conditions and is therefore routinely misdiagnosed. Following is a list of symptoms:

Head, Face, Neck
- Unexplained hair loss
- Headache, mild or severe, seizures
- Pressure in head, white matter lesions in brain (MRI)
- Twitching of facial or other muscles
- Facial paralysis (Bell's Palsy, Horner's syndrome)
- Tingling of nose, (tip of) tongue, cheek or facial flushing
- Stiff or painful neck
- Jaw pain or stiffness
- Dental problems
- Sore throat, clearing throat a lot, phlegm (flem), hoarseness, runny nose Eyes/Vision
- Double or blurry vision
- Increased floating spots
- Pain in eyes, or swelling around eyes
- Oversensitivity to light
- Flashing lights, peripheral waves or phantom images in corner of eyes Ears/Hearing
- Decreased hearing in one or both ears, plugged ears
- Buzzing in ears
- Pain in ears, over-sensitivity to sounds
- Ringing in one or both ears

Digestive and Excretory Systems
- Diarrhea
- Constipation
- Irritable bladder (trouble starting, stopping) or interstitial cystitis
- Upset stomach (nausea or pain) or GERD (gastroesophageal reflux disease) Musculoskeletal System
- Bone pain, joint pain or swelling, carpal tunnel syndrome
- Stiffness of joints, back, neck, tennis elbow
- Muscle pain or cramps, (Fibromyalgia)

Respiratory and Circulatory Systems

- Shortness of breath, can't get full/satisfying breath, cough
- Chest pain or rib soreness
- Night sweats or unexplained chills
- Heart palpitations or extra beats
- Endocarditis, heart blockage

Neurologic System
- Tremors or unexplained shaking
- Burning or stabbing sensations in the body
- Fatigue, Chronic Fatigue Syndrome, weakness, peripheral neuropathy or partial paralysis
- Pressure in the head
- Numbness in body, tingling, pinpricks
- Poor balance, dizziness, difficulty walking
- Increased motion sickness
- Light-headedness, wooziness

Psychological Well-being
- Mood swings, irritability, bi-polar disorder
- Unusual depression
- Disorientation (getting or feeling lost)
- Feeling as if you are losing your mind
- Over-emotional reactions, crying easily
- Too much sleep, or insomnia
- Difficulty falling or staying asleep
- Narcolepsy, sleep apnea
- Panic attacks, anxiety

Mental Capability
- Memory loss (short or long term)
- Confusion, difficulty thinking
- Difficulty with concentration or reading
- Going to the wrong place
- Speech difficulty (slurred or slow)
- Difficulty finding commonly used words
- Stammering speech
- Forgetting how to perform simple tasks

Reproduction and Sexuality
- Loss of sex drive
- Sexual dysfunction
- Unexplained menstrual pain, irregularity

- Unexplained breast pain, discharge
- Testicular or pelvic pain

General Well-being
- Phantom smells
- Unexplained weight gain or loss
- Extreme fatigue
- Swollen glands or lymph nodes
- Unexplained fevers (high or low grade)
- Continual infections (sinus, kidney, eye, etc.)
- Symptoms seem to change, come and go
- Pain migrates (moves) to different body parts
- Early on, experienced a "flu-like" illness, after which you have not since felt well
- Low body temperature
- Allergies or chemical sensitivities
- Increased effect from alcohol and possible worse hangover

Figure 3

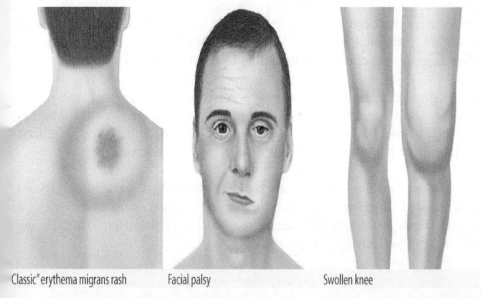

Classic" erythema migrans rash   Facial palsy   Swollen knee

1.3 A history of misdiagnosis and misinformation

As can be seen from the above list, Lyme is still one of the most misdiagnosed illnesses, hence the reason for both Lyme and Syphilis can be called The Great Imitator.

Patients with Lyme disease have been incorrectly diagnosed with: multiple sclerosis (MS), fibromyalgia, chronic fatigue syndrome, autoimmune diseases including lupus and rheumatoid arthritis [1-7] , polymyalgia rheumatica, thyroid disease and psychiatric disorders, among others.

Fatigue, insomnia, and myalgias are seen in both Fibromyalgia and Lyme disease. Chronic Fatigue Syndrome symptoms are often seen in Lyme disease patients and include severe fatigue, impaired memory and concentration, sleep disturbance, myalgias, and arthralgias.

Steere et al. described Lyme disease cases that were misdiagnosed as Juvenile Rheumatoid Arthritis (JRA). [8]

Nowakowski and Feder reported cases misdiagnosed as cellulitis. [9,10]
Plotkin described a 39-year-old male with a retropopliteal rash that progressed, within three weeks to Lyme disease, with a loss of consciousness and a complete heart block that required insertion of a transvenous cardiac pacemaker. [11]
Lyme disease has been mistaken for multiple sclerosis (MS). [12,13] In fact, one author estimated that 5% – 10% of patients presumed to have MS suffered from other conditions including Lyme disease. [14]

Three cases of neuroborreliosis were initially misdiagnosed as anterior ischemic optic neuropathy caused by giant cell arteritis. Neuropsychiatric presentations, including depression, anxiety and rage, have been identified in both acute and chronic Lyme disease cases. [15]

Lyme disease has also been mistaken for polymyalgia rheumatica [16,17], sports related injuries [18], and common medical conditions such as sinusitis, Epstein-Barr syndrome, rotator cuff tear, meniscus tear, edema, cellulitis, and pericarditis. [19].

Other misdiagnosis include:
Flu, Spider Bite, Allergic Hives,
Fibromyalgia, Multiple Sclerosis,
Hypochondria, Adolescent belligerence
Depression, Neurosis
Lupus
Other autoimmune & neurodegenerative
 diseases (Alzheimer's & Dementia)

Figure 4

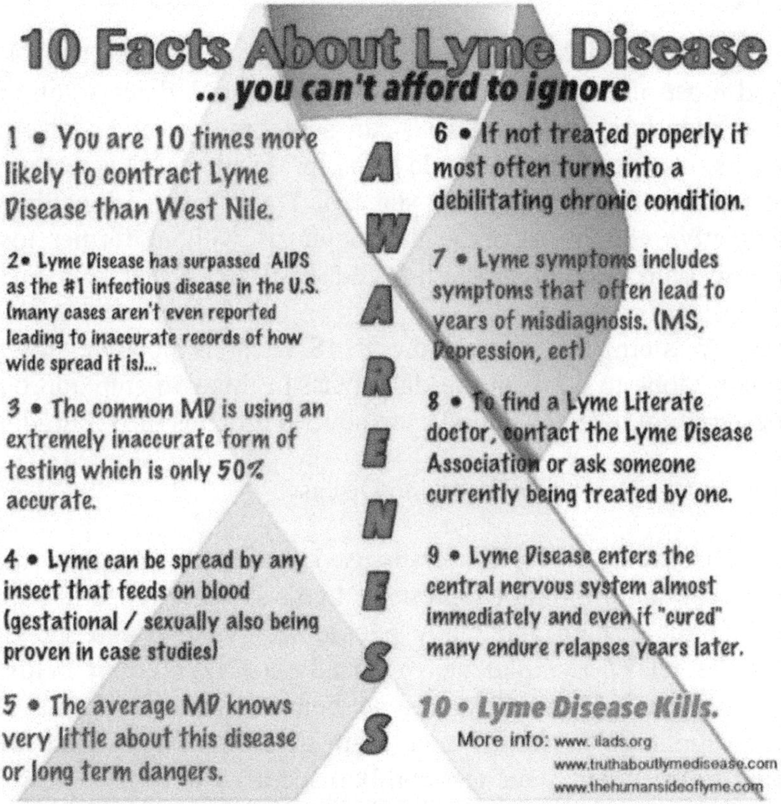

10 Facts About Lyme Disease
... you can't afford to ignore

1 • You are 10 times more likely to contract Lyme Disease than West Nile.

2• Lyme Disease has surpassed AIDS as the #1 infectious disease in the U.S. (many cases aren't even reported leading to inaccurate records of how wide spread it is)...

3 • The common MD is using an extremely inaccurate form of testing which is only 50% accurate.

4 • Lyme can be spread by any insect that feeds on blood (gestational / sexually also being proven in case studies)

5 • The average MD knows very little about this disease or long term dangers.

6 • If not treated properly it most often turns into a debilitating chronic condition.

7 • Lyme symptoms includes symptoms that often lead to years of misdiagnosis. (MS, Depression, ect)

8 • To find a Lyme Literate doctor, contact the Lyme Disease Association or ask someone currently being treated by one.

9 • Lyme Disease enters the central nervous system almost immediately and even if "cured" many endure relapses years later.

10 • Lyme Disease Kills.

More info: www.ilads.org
www.truthaboutlymedisease.com
www.thehumansideoflyme.com

AWARENESS

1.4   Current methods of diagnosis

The variable signs and symptoms of Lyme disease are nonspecific and often are found in other conditions, so diagnosis can be difficult. What's more, the ticks that transmit Lyme disease also can spread other diseases at the same time.

If you don't have the characteristic Lyme disease rash, your doctor might ask about your medical history, including whether you've been outdoors in the summer where Lyme disease is common, and do a physical exam.

Lab tests to identify antibodies to the bacteria can help confirm the diagnosis. These tests are most reliable a few weeks after an infection, after your body has had time to develop antibodies. They include:

- Enzyme-linked immunosorbent assay (ELISA) test. The test used most often to detect Lyme disease, ELISA detects antibodies to B. burgdorferi. But because it can sometimes provide false-positive results, it's not used as the sole basis for diagnosis. This test might not be positive during the early stage of Lyme disease, but the rash is distinctive enough to make the diagnosis without further testing in people who live in areas infested with ticks that transmit Lyme disease.
- Western blot test. If the ELISA test is positive, this test is usually done to confirm the diagnosis. In this two-step approach, the Western blot detects antibodies to several proteins of B. burgdorferi.

- CD57 Blood Test for Lyme Disease

The Lyme Disease CD57 HNK1 test is used to aid in the diagnosis of Lyme Disease as well as to monitor treatment. Lyme Disease tends to suppress a person's immune system and many people with Lyme have shown a low count for the CD57 Lymphocyte. Typically a CD57 count below 60 is indicative of Lyme Disease. In people being treated for Lyme Disease, monitoring their CD57 count can help determine how well they are responding to treatment. This test can be used as a screening, however not all Lyme people will show a lowered CD57 count and some conditions besides Lyme may lower this count as well. Confirmation with a Western Blot test is recommended.

1.5   Current methods of treatment

Early Lyme Disease

Lyme-literate doctors are likely to recommend more aggressive and longer antibiotic treatment for patients. They may, for instance, treat "high risk" tick bites where the tick came from an endemic area, was attached a long time, and was removed improperly. They may treat a Lyme rash for a longer period of time than the IDSA recommends, to ensure that the disease does not progress. They are unlikely to withhold treatment pending laboratory test results.

Late or Chronic Lyme Disease

Experts agree that the earlier you are treated the better, since early treatment is often successful. Unfortunately, a substantial portion of patients treated with short-term antibiotics continue to have significant symptoms. The quality of life of patients with chronic Lyme disease is similar to that of patients with congestive heart failure. Doctors don't agree about the cause of these ongoing symptoms. The primary cause of this debate is flawed diagnostic testing. There is currently no test that can determine whether a patient has active infection or whether the infection has been eradicated by treatment.

People treated with appropriate antibiotics in the early stages of Lyme disease usually recover rapidly and completely. Antibiotics commonly used for oral treatment include doxycycline, amoxicillin, or cefuroxime axetil. People with certain neurological or cardiac forms of illness may require intravenous treatment with antibiotics such as ceftriaxone or penicillin.

Treatment regimens listed in the following table are for localized (early) Lyme disease. See references below (Hu 2016; Sanchez 2016) for treatment of patients with disseminated (late) Lyme disease. These regimens are guidelines only and may need to be adjusted depending on a person's age, medical history, underlying health conditions, pregnancy status, or allergies.

Age Category	Drug	Dosage	Maximum	Duration, Days
Adults	Doxycycline	100 mg, twice per day orally	N/A	10-21*
	Cefuroxime axetil	500 mg, twice per day orally	N/A	14-21
	Amoxicillin	500 mg, three times per day orally	N/A	14-21
Children	Amoxicillin	50 mg/kg per day orally, divided into 3 doses	500 mg per dose	14-21
	Doxycycline	4 mg/kg per day orally, divided into 2 doses	100 mg per dose	10-21*
	Cefuroxime axetil	30 mg/kg per day orally, divided into 2 doses	500 mg per dose	14-21

Figure 5

19

Antibiotics are often used to treat Lyme disease. In general, recovery will be quicker and more complete the sooner treatment begins.

Antibiotics

- Oral antibiotics. These are the standard treatment for early-stage Lyme disease. These usually include doxycycline for adults and children older than 8, or amoxicillin or cefuroxime for adults, younger children, and pregnant or breast-feeding women. A 14- to 21-day course of antibiotics is usually recommended, but some studies suggest that courses lasting 10 to 14 days are equally effective.
- Intravenous antibiotics. If the disease involves the central nervous system, your doctor might recommend treatment with an intravenous antibiotic for 14 to 28 days. This is effective in eliminating infection, although it may take you some time to recover from your symptoms. Intravenous antibiotics can cause various side effects, including a lower white blood cell count, mild to severe diarrhea, or colonization or infection with other antibiotic-resistant organisms unrelated to Lyme.

After treatment, a small number of people still have some symptoms, such as muscle aches and fatigue. The cause of these continuing symptoms, known as post-treatment Lyme disease syndrome, is unknown, and treating with more antibiotics doesn't help. Some experts believe that certain people who get Lyme disease are predisposed to develop an autoimmune response that contributes to their symptoms. More research is needed.

Antibiotics can wipe out beneficial intestinal flora, leading to a wide variety of additional health problems. It is important to take probiotics while on antibiotics to maintain a healthy balance of gut bacteria.

Bismacine

The Food and Drug Administration warns against the use of bismacine, an injectable compound prescribed by some alternative medicine practitioners to treat Lyme disease. Bismacine, also known as chromacine, contains high levels of the metal bismuth. Although bismuth is safely used in some oral medications for stomach ulcers, it's not approved for use in injectable form or as a treatment for Lyme disease. Bismacine can cause bismuth poisoning, which may lead to heart and kidney failure.

Orthodox Treatments

Oral antibiotics are the first line of treatment for acute or early disseminated Lyme disease. They are the only proven protocol that effectively treats a Lyme infection. Ì All other treatments are experimental and should not be thought of as replacements for antibiotics. Commonly used antibiotics include: • doxycycline* • amoxicillin (use for children and pregnant women) • cefuroxime axetil • telithromycin

Five to 10 percent of patients treated with doxycycline or amoxicillin (14-30 days) do not respond to treatment (Smith et al 2002). This may be due to co-infections or other unknown factors. * Will also treat ehrlichiosis, STARI, Rocky Mountain spotted fever, human granulocytic anaplasmosis

Intravenous antibiotics are usually used for neurological symptoms and chronic arthralgia associated with PLDS. These include: • ceftriaxone (use five days on, two to three days off to prevent cholecystitis) • benzathine penicillin (can be administered intramuscular or intravenous) • cefotaxime • doxycycline

Oral antibiotics are usually administered for two to four weeks. Some Lyme specialists continue medication at least four to six weeks and combine two to three different types of antibiotics in a protocol for persistent Lyme disease. Intravenous antibiotics are administered at least four to six months, even though there are no studies confirming the effectiveness of this therapy beyond a sixweek time frame. The common side effects associated with oral antibiotics include nausea, diarrhea, sun sensitivity, vaginal yeast infections, rash, glossitis, and abdominal pain. The use of probiotics with fructo-oligosaccharides (FOS) during antibiotic treatment can reduce many of the digestive yeast overgrowth and antibiotic related colitis (Clostridium difficile) side effects associated with antibiotic use. Many of the IV antibiotics require a central line, as they are caustic and they frequently cause a Jarisch Herxheimer-like reaction in patients.

A review by Warshafsky et al suggests that if a prophylactic antibiotic is given within 72 hours of a tick bite, it is effective for preventing transmission of Lyme disease (Warshafsky et al 2010). In the original study (Nadelman 2001) a single 200-mg dose of doxycycline prevented patients from developing Lyme disease 87 percent of the time compared to placebo. Readers should be aware that even with the placebo, transmission rates were surprisingly low. Most Lyme specialists would strongly advise against using this type of abrogated therapy.

In persistent Lyme disease, the use of steroids and other immuno-suppressive medications should be absolutely avoided as they contribute to the progression of this illness and will likely cause treatment failure. Lack of sleep, alcohol use (except for small amounts in tinctures), cigarette smoking, and nutrient deficiencies can also contribute to poor patient response.

Why Antibiotics May Not Work for Lyme Disease
- Borrelia burgdorferi, the bacteria that causes Lyme disease, has a corkscrew shape that allows it to bore deep into tissues and cartilage (including the brain and nervous system), safely out of reach of most antibiotics.
- Borrelia burgdorferi can give up its corkscrew shape and convert to a form that is able to live inside cells ("intracellular") where again, antibiotics have less reach.
- Borrelia burgdorferi, along with other similar microbes, can form dormant cysts that are completely resistant to antibiotics; the harder you hit it, the more resistant it becomes.
- Borrelia burgdorferi is usually accompanied and aided by co-infections of other stealth microbes that also live inside cells.

Antibiotic resistance occurs at a high rate with these types of microbes. An antibiotic is one single chemical substance. Bacteria, such as Borrelia (and also its co-infections), respond slowly to antibiotics and have more time to develop resistance to the antibiotic. In other words, the longer they can hang on, the more likely they are to become completely antibiotic resistant. Using multiple antibiotics at once seems to accelerate this process and alternating antibiotics doesn't seem to help. Resistant bacteria become even more entrenched.

Antibiotics destroy the normal flora (friendly bacteria) in the gut and skin, causing bacterial imbalance and a host of other symptoms in the body. Most importantly, use of antibiotics suppresses immune function, which may present the greatest hurdle to recovery—you cannot get well without optimal immune function.

Borrelia burgdorferi can exist in biofilms, which are protected colonies of microbes that form on a surface (such as plaque on your teeth), but what role this plays in Lyme disease is controversial. The symptom profile of Lyme disease suggests that it is not a biofilm disease and that biofilms are not a big factor in overcoming Lyme.

CHAPTER 2

Holistic Protocols

Natural treatment options for Lyme disease are often more effective than antibiotics and prescription medication. Tweaking the daily diet as well as supplementing one's daily routine often relieve the symptoms of Lyme disease and naturally cure the condition. Small changes like exercising, taking probiotics and adding herbs to a daily routine destroys Lyme bacteria in the body and reduces symptoms.

Your Gut and Your immune System

Chronic infection is an underlying factor in most chronic illnesses. Our sugar-laden diet, GMO foods that kill beneficial bacteria, antibiotics, other antibacterial products, and many of the chemicals in our food supply deplete our beneficial bacteria, which wreaks havoc on our immune systems. This sets the stage for systemic, chronic fungal infections and parasites to multiply, permeate the gut, enter the body's bloodstream, and spread infection throughout the body.

Conventional doctors are very bad at finding and diagnosing parasitical and fungal infections that cannot easily be seen on the surface of the body. The average person is dealing with Candida overgrowth at the very least (the most common fungal infection in our bodies) due to the aforementioned modern diet and lifestyle.

Obviously, to treat a difficult bacterial infection such as Lyme (or whatever combination of bacteria, viruses, and parasites causing Lyme symptoms) the immune system needs to be as strong as possible. The immune system is only as healthy as the gut. The body's intestinal tract mirrors the body's health and dictates the power of the immune system. Step one is to balance the gut flora and eliminate most of the harmful pathogens in the body.

Diet

A healthy diet relies on a foundation of on raw, fresh, organic (when possible), whole foods and herbs. A vegan diet has proven over an over again as the most optimal diet for supplying the body the micro-nutrients need to support the immune system. Salads are one of the best ways to do this. Not your typical iceberg lettuce salads with a few carrots shreds and some ranch dressing, but a salad with a wide variety of at least 10 different vegetables along with fresh garlic, turmeric, ginger, unrefined sea salt, and healthy fats. It is the best way to get a wide array of the best nutrients that will repair the gut and rebuild the body's immune system. Don't underestimate this; a large salad every day, done right, will do more for the body than any supplement regimen, and when followed long enough, the right diet with these kinds of daily salads can completely heal the body from disease, in most cases. But the right supplement protocol can radically speed things up and is often necessary for the very ill.

A perfect diet would not be complete without lots of clean drinking water. For detoxification, cranberry Stevia lemonade is very good for rejuvenating the kidneys, cleaning the liver, purifying blood, and flushing out the whole system. For most people, a gallon a day will yield remarkable results, but for smaller people, or those who have rare conditions that make this dangerous, use common sense and don't ever drink too much water (or any fluid). And for everyone else, a gallon of cranberry lemonade every day will have amazing benefits, second only to salads and cutting out other junk food, but again, use common sense. Drinking that much water in a very short period of time can kill people, believe it or not.

Lifestyle Remedies for Tick-Borne Illness
If caught early enough, Lyme disease can typically be treated using several lifestyle remedies. Regular exercise augments the amount of oxygen in the body and blood, which acts to destroy the Lyme bacteria in the blood. Additionally, probiotics taken daily boosts the number of good bacteria in the gut, supplementing the immune system.

Herbal Treatment for Lyme

Certain herbs have also been shown to suppress microbial threats like Lyme disease. Andrographis, cat's claw and sarsaparilla constitute three of the most important Lyme disease treatment options. These herbs effectively suppress Lyme bacteria with limited side effects or reactions.

Andrographis

An antiviral and antibacterial herb, andrographis has proven to also have patristic properties. Often used in treatment for common viral illnesses, this herb delivers a variety

of healing properties. Regular dosing of this herb delivers liver protection, immune enhancement and cardiovascular benefits, making it a good addition to a Lyme disease fighting regimen.

Cat's Claw

Known for its treatment of microbial conditions, cat's claw is an herb used primarily in treating Lyme disease. The herb offers several healing properties including antiparisitic, anti-inflammatory and antioxidant benefits.

Sarsaparilla

An antibacterial herb, sarsaparilla is particularly effective for treating infection. Additionally, it delivers anti-inflammatory properties and antioxidant benefits. Sarsaparilla is a safe, natural Lyme disease cure.

Early detection is key to successful treatment of Lyme. However, following a strict, natural treatment regimen can offer extensive benefits at any stage of the disease.

Alternatives for Treating Persistent Lyme Disease Syndrome (PLDS)

Many patients with PLDS are highly resistant to treatment. There are several causes for this. First, the Borrelia burgdorferi (Bb) organism can be found in blood and intercellular fluids as well as muscle, nerve, and organ tissue. No single antibiotic is effective for treating infections disseminated in both bodily fluids and various tissues. Secondly, Bb is pleomorphic and can exist in at least two and possibly three forms (Miklossy et al 2008). The L-form, or spheroplast, has no cell wall and is not susceptible to the same types of antibiotics as is the spirochete. A third possible form, a cyst form, is controversial, but may be able to lie dormant during conventional treatment and they cannot be killed by most antibiotics. Metronidazole and tinidazole are recommended (Burrascano 2008).

The following protocol has been used with some success in patients with PLDS that had previously been treated with oral and intravenous antibiotics. Most of these patients were symptom-free as long as they continued intravenous antibiotics, but for various reasons (especially cost) they were unable to continue with that therapy. Of the 150+ patients that I have treated using various incarnations of this protocol (several hundred people under the supervision of other clinicians have also been treated with my protocol), approximately 65 percent are symptom free or have greatly reduced symptoms; 20 percent showed moderate improvement, and 15 percent did not respond. A larger, well-designed study is needed to substantiate these clinical findings.

Herbal Therapy

Lyme Formula #1: Spirolyd Compound™ (by Herbalist & Alchemist) Dosage: 3-4 ml TID. Take for two weeks before adding in the Spirolyd Support™ formula. Patients with gastritis or gastric ulcers should take with food to prevent further GI irritation.

• Sarsaparilla rhizome (Smilax spp.) –traditional syphilis treatment; anti-inflammatory; alterative • Guaiac resin (Guaiacum officinale) – traditional syphilis treatment; anti-inflammatory; antibacterial • Stillingia root (Stillingia sylvatica) – traditional syphilis treatment; clears blood heat; alterative • Andrographis herb (Andrographis paniculata) – clears blood heat (infections); antiamoebic, antibacterial and hepatoprotective

• Prickly ash bark (Zanthoxylum clava-herculis) –antibacterial and antiviral; relieves bone pain and arthralgia; enhances circulation and absorption

Lyme Formula #2: Spirolyd Support™ by Herbalist & Alchemist Dosage: 2-4 ml TID. Take concurrently with Spirolyd Compound™ for two weeks, then discontinue for two weeks, then reintroduce for two weeks. This pattern should be continued throughout treatment.

The rationale for this second formula is that the Borrelia spirochete can become resistant to treatment if the same antibiotic or herb is used. The addition of the second formula is designed to prevent resistance, which supposedly with herbs should not occur, but clinically seems to happen in some cases.

• Houttuynia herb (Houttuynia cordata) – clears blood heat (infections); antibacterial, antiviral and antifungal • Teasel root (Dipsacus asper) – anti-inflammatory; helps relieve arthralgia • Boneset herb (Eupatorium perfoliatum) –diaphoretic, antibacterial and immunostimulant; relieves bone and muscle pain • Isatis root (Isatis indigotica) –antibacterial and antiviral; clears blood heat (infections) • Lomatium root (Lomatium dissectum) –antibacterial, antiviral and antifungal

Note: The herbs alone are not effective to resolve Lyme disease (except for in canines).

Heat Therapy

Daily elevation of core body temperature to 101.5 to 102 degrees Fahrenheit, once per day for 15 minutes, inhibits Borrelia reproduction and enhances effectiveness of the herbal or antibiotic treatment (Reisengcr 1996). Take care to hydrate the patient and replace lost minerals, especially calcium, magnesium and zinc.

Saunas, hot tubs, and steam baths are probably the most effective methods for elevating body temperature. If not available, hot baths combined with taking a diaphoretic tea [yarrow (Achillea millefolium), elderflower (Sambucus nigra), ginger (Zingiber officinale)] can be substituted.

Note: Fever therapy alone is not effective to resolve Lyme disease.

These therapies together show greater activity than either one alone. Combining the use of the herbs and elevation of body temperature with antibiotic therapy results in improved outcomes over antibiotics alone or alternative therapies alone.

Other Proposed "Cures" for Lyme Disease

Teasel root (Dipsacus fullonum) – Some herbalists claim to have had success treating Lyme disease with very small doses of the common weedy teasel root. My clinical experience with this herb has confirmed that it is effective for relieving joint pain (Lyme arthralgia), but I have not been able to duplicate their experience in resolving confirmed cases of Lyme disease with my patients. I prefer to use the Asian xu duan (D. asper, D. japonica) as it seems to me to be more effective and less likely to cause nausea and digestive upset.

Spilanthes (Spilanthes acmella) is claimed by some practitioners to have antibacterial activity, especially against spirochetes. I know of no published data to support this claim. The herb does have antibacterial, antifungal, and immunostimulating effects.

Cat's claw bark (Uncaria tomentosa, U. guianensis) – A small study (28 people) was done comparing a tetracyclic oxindole alkaloid- (TOA) free cat's claw product with antibiotic therapy. Reportedly, 85 percent of the cat's claw group (14 people) were seronegative after six months for Bb and had dramatic improvement in their symptoms. The control group treated with antibiotics fared poorly. This study by Cowden, W., Moayad, H., et al, is available as a preliminary report on the Internet (http://www.samento.com.ec/sciencelib/sarticles/Studyshowssamento.htm) and has never been published as far as I can tell. There are many questions about the study's validity. In addition, the whole TOA and pentacyclic oxindole alkaloid (POA) controversy concerning Uncaria is false and based on marketing rather than science. Cat's claw does clear blood heat (infections) and may be of some benefit for treating Lyme disease, but in clinical practice when used by itself it has not produced dramatic improvements in most people that I have treated.

Japanese knotweed root (Polygonum cuspidatum) – Many websites promote this herb as a "cure" for Lyme disease. It is useful for treating Lyme arthralgia (Damp-Heat arthritis) and is a rich source of resveratrol, which is an effective antioxidant and anti-inflammatory. While the root has antibacterial activity and can be a useful part of a Lyme protocol, I do not believe it is a cure for Lyme disease.

Homeopathic ledum (Ledum palustre) is recommended to prevent and treat Lyme disease. It is also widely used in the veterinary community to treat canine and equine cases. While anecdotal stories of Lyme "cures" and improvements abound, there are no studies that I am aware of showing this treatment is effective.

Herbal/Nutritional Protocols for Lyme Disease Symptoms

Muscle and neck pain or spasm

• Ashwagandha root (Withania somnifera) is an adaptogen, antispasmodic and anxiolytic useful for muscle or fibromyalgia pain. • Black cohosh root (Actaea racemosa) is an antispasmodic and analgesic used for muscle pain. Do not use it with hepatotoxic antibiotics. • Blue vervain herb (Verbena hastata) is effective for muscle spasms and facial tics that are exacerbated by stress. Use it with carminatives to prevent nausea. • Siler/Ledebouriella, fang feng root (Saposhnikovia divaricata) is effective for treating Liver Wind muscle spasms or migratory pain. • Gambir, gou teng thorns (Uncaria sinensis) have antispasmodic and analgesic activity and are used to treat spasms, facial and neck pain. • Kava root (Piper methysticum) is an effective muscle antispasmodic, analgesic and anxiolytic. Do not use it with hepatotoxic antibiotics. • Kudzu root (Pueraria lobata) is used to relieve muscle spasms, stiff neck, or sore, achy muscles. • Magnesium, 400-600 mg per day, is effective for treating muscle spasms, restless leg syndrome and facial tics. Take either liquid magnesium or the L-lactate dihydrate form. Topical magnesium gels also seem to be effective. • Skullcap herb (Scutellaria lateriflora) is a nervine for patients who develop nervous tics, tremors, palsies, and spasms under stress. It is also of benefit for headaches where the scalp muscles are sore. • Wood betony herb (Pedicularis spp.) is used for muscles that feel tired, overworked, and sore.

Lyme arthralgia (joint pain)

• Ba ji tian root (Morinda officinalis) is used for knee, ankle, and low back pain. It is also an antidepressant and may have mild adaptogenic effects. • Glucosamine (500 mg-1000 mg) with MSM (500 mg) BID/TID is useful for painful joints and arthritic pain. It has anti-inflammatory activity. • Japanese knotweed root, hu zhang (Polygonum cuspidatum) clears Damp-Heat and WindDamp conditions with blood stasis and pain. It is useful for Lyme arthralgia and contains resveratrol, which is a potent antioxidant and anti-inflammatory. • Huai niu xi root (Achyranthes bidentata) is used in Traditional Chinese Medicine (TCM) for painful tendons, ligaments, and joints. • Solomon's seal root (Polygonatum biflorum) is especially useful for joint, disc, and cartilage pain and injuries. • Teasel root, xu duan (Dipsacus asper) is an effective anti-inflammatory for painful joints, tendons, and ligaments and it significantly helps Lyme arthralgia. • Coix seed, yi yi ren (Coix lachryma-jobi) increases joint mobility, has anti-inflammatory activity and relieves muscle spasms.

General Anti-inflammatories for Lyme arthralgia

• Alpha lipoic acid is useful for Lyme-induced peripheral neuropathy. It also promotes Co-Q-10 absorption and improves antioxidant status (250 mg BID). • Blueberry fruit (Vaccinium spp.) is a nutritive anti-inflammatory which benefits visual and cognitive problems and reduces allergic response. • Boswellia gum (Boswellia serrata) is a warming anti-inflammatory, analgesic and antifungal agent. • Cat's claw bark (Uncaria tomentosa, U. guianensis) is an immunomodulator and cooling antiinflammatory. It heals the gut mucosa and is useful for leaky gut syndrome. • Chai hu root (Bupleurum chinensis) is a cooling anti-inflammatory, hepatoprotective and antibacterial agent. I use it for migratory pain caused by Lyme disease. • EPA/DHA (Omega 3 flax oils) are anti-inflammatory and reduce inflammatory prostaglandin production (4-6 g per day). • Ginger rhizome (Zingiber officinale) is a warming anti-inflammatory and carminative. • Sarsaparilla rhizome (Smilax spp.) is a cooling anti-inflammatory. It binds endotoxins in the gut, enhancing their excretion, and may be useful for promoting excretion of Babesia hemotoxins. • Turmeric rhizome (Curcuma longa) is hepatoprotective, a warming anti-inflammatory, and it heals the gut mucosa. • Yucca root (Yucca spp.) is a cooling anti-inflammatory used for arthritic pain.

Neurological and cognitive symptoms including poor memory, lack of concentration, and confusion • Acetyl-L-carnitine can help improve cognitive function, mood and memory (1500-2000 mg per day). • Bacopa herb (Bacopa monnieri) is an anxiolytic, nootropic, nervine and thyroid stimulant. • Ginkgo standardized extract (Ginkgo biloba) is a cerebral stimulant, antioxidant and it inhibits platelet activating factor (PAF). • Gotu kola herb (Centella asiatica) is a cerebral stimulant, anti-inflammatory and anxiolytic.

   • Holy basil (Ocimum tenuiflorum) is a mild adaptogen, cerebral stimulant, antioxidant, and antibacterial. • Lemon balm herb (Melissa officinalis) is a nervine, antibacterial and carminative. • Rhodiola root (Rhodiola rosea) is a stimulating adaptogen, antidepressant and antioxidant. • Rosemary herb (Rosmarinus officinalis) is a cerebral stimulant, antibacterial and carminative. • St. John's wort flowering herb (Hypericum perforatum) is a nervine, antidepressant and antiinflammatory. It is also used for nerve pain. • Schisandra berry, wu wei zi (Schisandra chinensis) is an adaptogen, nootropic, hepatoprotective agent and antioxidant. It is calming and provides a feeling of alertness and increased focus. • White peony root, bai shao (Paeonia lactiflora) enhances cognitive function, is a nootropic and it relieves brain fog caused by deficient blood.

Bell's palsy • Mullein root (Verbascum thapsus) is specific for facial nerve pain and inflammation. • Prickly ash bark (Zanthoxylum spp.) is a circulatory stimulant and it relieves peripheral nerve pain. • St. John's wort flowering tops (Hypericum perforatum) is useful for nerve pain and inflammation. • Sub-lingual B-12 (methylcobalamin form only) often works in three to seven days to relieve Bell's palsy (1 mg/day). • Sweet melilot herb (Melilotus alba or M. officinalis) is indicated for sharp, stabbing nerve pain.

Lyme insomnia • Biota seed, bai zi ren (Platycladus orientalis) calms disturbed Shen and is useful for treating insomnia, anxiety, fear, night sweats, and cardiac palpitations. • Gambir, gou teng thorns (Uncaria sinensis) are useful for irritability and anxiety inhibiting sleep. • Hops strobiles (Humulus lupulus) are sedative, anxiolytic and analgesic. • Passionflower herb (Passiflora incarnata) is a nervine/sedative, relieves circular thinking, and occipital headaches. • Ye jiao teng stem (Polygonum multiflorum) calms disturbed Shen; use with jujube seed and passionflower for insomnia, anxiety and nightmares. • Jujube seed, suan zao ren (Zizyphus spinosa) calms disturbed Shen and is effective for treating insomnia, nightmares, palpitations, and anxiety.

Lyme anxiety • Bacopa herb (Bacopa monnieri) is an anxiolytic, nootropics and nervine. • Blue vervain herb (Verbena hastata) is an anxiolytic and it helps control muscle spasms and nervous tics. • Chinese Polygala root, yuan zhi (Polygala tenuifolia) is a strong anxiolytic and sedative. • Fresh oat (Avena sativa) is a nervine and mild anxiolytic for people who are emotionally brittle or highly labile. • Motherwort herb (Leonurus cardiaca) is an anxiolytic and nervine, it helps controls cardiac palpitations. • Pulsatilla herb (Anemone patens) is a strong anxiolytic used for panic attacks. It is toxic in overdose.

• Ye jiao teng stem (Polygonum multiflorum) calms disturbed Shen, use it with jujube seed and passionflower for insomnia, anxiety and nightmares.

Fatigue and HPA axis depletion • American ginseng root (Panax quinquefolius) is a nourishing adaptogen and immune amphoteric. • Ashwagandha root (Withania somnifera) is a calming adaptogen, especially if the patient has hypothyroid function and low hemoglobin. It is also an immune amphoteric. • Asian ginseng root, ren shen (Panax ginseng) is a stimulating adaptogen, anti-inflammatory and immune amphoteric. Red ginseng is most appropriate for people who are cold, deficient and exhausted. • Co-Q-10 (Ubiquinone) enhances energy and oxygenation of tissues (100 mg TID). • Cordyceps fungus, dong chong xia cao (Cordyceps chinensis) nourishing adaptogen, immune amphoteric. It also has hepato- and nephroprotective activity. • Eleuthero root (Eleutherococcus senticosus) is a mild adaptogen, immune amphoteric and antioxidant. • Holy basil herb (Ocimum tenuiflorum) is a mild adaptogen, nootropic and immune amphoteric. • Rhodiola root (Rhodiola rosea) is a stimulating adaptogen, antidepressant, antioxidant and cardiac tonic. • Schisandra berry, wu wei zi

(Schisandra chinensis) is a calming adaptogen, hepatoprotective, antioxidant and immune amphoteric.

Immunodeficiency in persistent Lyme disease: • Astragalus root, huang qi (Astragalus membranaceus) is an immune amphoteric and it has cardioprotective and nephroprotective activity. • Cat's claw bark (Uncaria tomentosa, U. guianensis) is an immune amphoteric and antibacterial agent. • Chaga sclerotium (Inonotus obliquus) is an immunopotentiator. • Maitake mushroom (Grifola frondosa) is an immune amphoteric. • Reishi mushroom, ling zhi (Ganoderma sinensis) is an immune amphoteric and mild calming adaptogen. • Also see adaptogens under Fatigue.

To prevent liver damage due to the use of potentially hepatotoxic antibiotics [tetracycline, cefriaxone, atovaquone (used for babesiosis), minocycline, and high-dose doxycycline]: • Standardized milk thistle seed (Silybum marianum) is hepatoprotective, antioxidant and antiinflammatory. • Schisandra berry, wu wei zi (Schisandra chinensis) is hepatoprotective, antioxidant and antiinflammatory. • Turmeric (Curcuma longa) is hepatoprotective, antioxidant and anti-inflammatory.

Herbs used to help prevent yeast overgrowth from long-term antibiotic use: • Berberine-containing herbs are antifungal, they include goldenseal (Hydrastis canadensis), Chinese coptis (huang lian, Coptis chinensis), Oregon grape root (Mahonia spp.), barberry (Berberis spp.), yellow root (Xanthorhiza simpliccisima). • Cardamom seed (Elettaria cardamomum) is antifungal and inhibits Candida albicans. It is also antibacterial. • Fireweed herb (Epilobium angustifolium) is antifungal and inhibits Candida albicans.
  • Garlic bulb (Allium sativum) is antifungal and inhibits Candida albicans. It also has antibacterial activity. • Spilanthes herb (Spilanthes acmella) is antifungal and inhibits Candida albicans. It also has antibacterial activity. • Probiotics and fermented foods help prevent depletion of normal healthy bowel and vaginal flora and inhibit overgrowth of pathogenic bacteria, fungi and yeast.

2.1   My Protocols to date

In my 20 years of practice I have found a holistic program to be much more effective in treating chronic diseases such as Lyme disease than the currently accepted protocols with conventional medicine. As holistic implies, this utilizes cleansing protocols, dietary, nutrition and lifestyle changes, herbal medicine, exercise, fresh air, etc. I have found if patients consistently follow the program as laid out we have found a very high success rate with the Lyme bacteria undetectable in the blood along with cessation of the collateral damage caused by the original infection. In this section I will layout the protocol, step by step as I have used it in my practice.

TIME LINE:

With most cases, I have seen cures for chronic Lyme normally taking anywhere from nine months to a year, depending on the severity of the case as well as the commitment of the patient. A cure is defined as the following:

a.) No live Borrilis bacteria is detectable in the blood.
b.) The CD57 is 200 and above.
c.) Any sign co-infections is not longer present in the blood.
d.) All previous symptoms of chronic Lyme have been eliminated.
Acute Lyme, meaning the patient has not been infected for any longer than three months, we have seen the above definition of a cure averaging three months.

2.2 CANDIDA CLEANSE:

The first step in my program is to aid the patient in returning the immune system back to a state where it can begin to fight the disease. Since one of the most common disorders affecting the immune system in this country is a candida overgrowth, we start with a cleanse to purge the body of excess of candida and begin to re-establish the micro-flora environment.

Definition of a Candida Overgrowth

The perforated bowel is referred to as Leaky Gut Syndrome. This condition also allows undigested protein to enter the bloodstream. These proteins are foreign to the immune system and are therefore attacked. The immune system remembers these protein invaders and reacts like an allergy each time you consume them. This opens up the possibility of eventually making you allergic to every food you eat.

Since yeast overgrowth can cause symptoms mimicking many diseases, misdiagnosis is common and yeast overgrowth remains undetected allowing it to further colonize, thus creating more side effects and ill health. Many people have suffered for decades going from doctor to doctor, therapy to therapy and eventually being prescribed anti-depressants from doctors who are incapable of a proper diagnosis, so they determine that it is in the head of the patients. This incompetence on the part of modern medicine hopefully leads these unfortunate patients to alternative therapy.

Most alternative therapy focuses on killing off the yeast and providing the body with the pro- biotics. These therapies fail to correct the damaged intestinal tract which allows the yeast condition to return. The following twenty day protocol addresses all aspects of treatment and can permanently eliminate Systemic Yeast Overgrowth and Leaky Gut Syndrome.

First procedure: On the first two days consume two quarts of a decoction of Black Walnut and Pau d' arco (one quart each day). This is made by simmering the herbs in water for twenty minutes at the rate of one tablespoon of the combined herbs (equal parts) per cup of water. An easier alternative would be to take five capsules five times a day of Dr. Christopher's Intestinal Sweep Formula. This procedure will kill off the yeast, which on other programs can make you feel very nauseous. This

36

nauseous feeling is avoided by taking plant-based digestive enzymes in large amounts (triple the stated dosages on the label) and flushing out with Dr. Christopher's Lower Bowel formula during these first two days. NOTES: The Lower Bowel formula can be taken the whole time if needed. You should have 3 bowels movements a day and the amount of Lower Bowel taken is the amount needed to give you 3 bowel movements a day. It is most important during that first procedure so that the body is eliminating the yeast etc. Udo's Choice has plant-based digestive enzymes, which are available at most herb shops.

Second procedure: For the next 14 days, take five capsules five times per day of Dr. Christopher's Soothing Digestion formula, or one tablespoon of slippery elm gruel five times a day. Either of these methods will coat, soothe and heal the lesions in the intestinal wall. (You can continue to take the Intestinal Sweep Formula 2 capsules 3 times a day during this time.)

Third procedure: For the next two days repeat the first procedure.

Fourth procedure: Take copious (triple the stated dosages on the label) amounts of multi-strain Pro- biotics to re-establish the flora. Further aids would be to eat raw sauerkraut, Kim Chi, raw apple cider vinegar, Rejuvelac, or miso in large amounts, which are the exact foods to stay away from if you have leaky gut syndrome, yet they rebuild the flora once the leaky gut is healed. NOTES: Udo's Choice has Pro-biotics, are available at most herb shops. The pro-biotics need to be taken for about a week to rebuild the flora. Note: It is absolutely essential that you do not feed the yeast during this procedure. Therefore, do not consume any sugar or alcohol in any form. This includes all dairy, grains, and fruit. This is twenty days of a wonderful vegetable, nuts, seeds and sprouted legume diet; thus insuring a healthy life, free of Systemic Yeast Overgrowth.

Candida/Leaky Gut Syndrome Cleanse Schedule						
IS = Intestinal Sweep	LB = Lower Bowel		SD = Soothing Digestion			

	Date	7:00am	10:00am	1:00pm	4:00pm	7:00pm
Step 1 2 DAYS Intestinal Sweep IS=50 LB=12		5-IS/2-LB	5-IS	5-IS/2-LB	5-IS	5-IS/2-LB
	1					
	2					

		7:00am	10:00am	1:00pm	4:00pm	7:00pm
		5-SD/2-IS	5-SD	5-SD/2-IS	5-SD	5-SD/2-IS
	3					
	4					
	5					
	6					
Step 2 14 DAYS Soothing Digestion SD=350 13 DAYS Intestinal Sweep IS= 78	7					
	8					
	9					
	10					
	11					
	12					
	13					
	14					
	15					
	16					

		7:00am	10:00am	1:00pm	4:00pm	7:00pm
Step 3 2 DAYS Intestinal Sweep IS=50 LB=12		5-IS/2-LB	5-IS	5-IS/2-LB	5-IS	5-IS/2-LB
	17					
	18					

		7:00am	10:00am	1:00pm	4:00pm	7:00pm
	Select Probiotic of Choice	*Probiotics	*Probiotics	*Probiotics	*Probiotics	*Probiotics
Step 4 2 MOS Re-establish Flora: *Probiotics 3x label dosage or Large Amounts of: *Raw Sauerkraut *Kim Chi *Raw Apple Cider Vinegar *Rejuvelac *Miso	19					

Herbs required: 2 Bottles-Soothing Digestion 1 Bottle-Intestinal Sweep 1 Bottle-Lower Bowel

Notes: You should have 3 bowel movements a day. This is most important during the first procedure so that the body is eliminating the yeast, etc... If necessary, the Lower Bowel formula can be taken the entire time. In some cases, a colonic might be necessary.

Figure 6

CANDIDA MENU PLAN

Monday
Breakfast: Oatmeal(using the thermos method) with almond milk(unsweetened) add tsp of cinnamon Sprinkle on some hulled hemp seeds.
Midmorning: juice with celery, parsley, and spinach
Lunch: salad with mixed greens, cucumber with garlic, lemon, olive and flax oil dressing. 1 carrot and 1celery stick. Hand full of walnuts.
Dinner: Tempeh or Tofu (organic or GMO free) stir fry with brown rice and tahini sauce, grilled/baked vegetables (zucchini, onion, garlic, and squash) green salad with a garlic, lemon and olive oil dressing.

Tuesday
Breakfast: Oatmeal(using the thermos method) with almond milk(unsweetened) add tsp of cinnamon
Midmorning: juice with cucumber, 1 carrot, parsley
Lunch: Green salad or bean salad (no sugar), avocado, green onion with garlic and oil, grilled vegetables
Dinner: Vegan Sushi rolls(use brown rice only) made with avocado, carrot and mushroom. Green salad made with Tahini dressing and sunflower seeds)

Wednesday
Breakfast: Oatmeal(using the thermos method) with almond milk(unsweetened) add tsp of cinnamon
Midmorning: juice with celery, parsley, and mixed greens
Lunch: Green salad with spinach, sunflower seeds, cucumber, with garlic, lemon, ginger and olive oil dressing.
Dinner: vegan pattie on 2 slices of Ezekiel bread or Vegetable Quinoa, Add slice of tomato, Mushrooms, onion with 2 carrot and celery sticks. Green salad with tahini dressing.

Thursday
Breakfast: Oatmeal(using the thermos method) with almond milk(unsweetened) add tsp of cinnamon.
Midmorning: juice with cucumber, parsley, and spinach
Lunch: Green salad with cabbage, green onion, 1/2 grated carrot, with ginger, oil, lemon, garlic, and dill for dressing, hand full of walnuts.

Dinner: grilled or steamed vegetables over brown rice. Sliced tomato 1 slice of Ezekiel bread. Hummus with radishes or celery.

Friday

Breakfast: Oatmeal(using the thermos method) with almond milk(unsweetened) add tsp of cinnamon.

Midmorning: juice with celery, parsley.

Lunch: salad with Romaine Lettuce, avocado, green onion with Garlic and oil dressing, black bean soup with grilled vegetables

Dinner: Vegan burger sandwich(see above on what to add) or Vegetable Quinoa with a green salad or Sushi rolls.

You can also snack on black bean soup, parsley soup, and vegetable broth in rotation. It is fine to mix and match.

The above menu plan is an example. Mondays do not have be Monday, Tuesdays do not have to be Tuesday. You can mix and swap individual meals. Also, the weekend, Saturday and Sunday, also use the same meals. The most important thing to take from this is if it (food) is on the menu plan, you can eat it. If it is not, than you cannot. You are attempting to starve the candida while the holistic medications eradicate it.

If you like you can add PLAIN(NOSUGAR) plant yogurt to any of the days. Maybe have a cup for breakfast instead of Oatmeal or add it with the oatmeal.

      **For your yogurt you can add a few walnuts or sunflower seeds.

      **Hummous can be used on the vegan burgers or use as a dressing.

DIETARY/NUTRITION:

Once the candida cleanse is done, the patient is then instructed to follow a strict but diverse vegan diet. This is duet o t several reasons. This allows for a significantly reduced mucous-less diet raising the pH of the patient and allowing less mucous for the bacteria to feed upon. It also drastically lowers the arachidonic acid levels. Lowering this EFA has been found to dramatically decrease the amount of systemic inflammation, thereby lowering the level of joint pain in the patient, a very common symptom of Lyme.

Part of the program entails nutrition education whereby we supply the patient with vegan menu plans, nutrition charts detailing foods high in protein, calcium, magnesium, potassium and other naturally occurring vitamins and minerals.

MEDICATION (STANDARD AMONGST ALL PATIENTS):
Holistic medication is second to nutrition in this program. As I tell the patients, holistic medications can work very well but they have ot have something, building blocks, to work with and that comes from nutrition. One of the first assessments for a proper Lyme program is to ascertain the patient's list of symptoms, which then enables the practitioner to define some of the collateral damage done by the disease. In most case, this presents as joint and muscle pain, nerve damage, heart issues if they have had the disease for a significantly long period of time, fatigue, and malnutrition.

We start all Lyme patients with a standard list of holistic medications (herbal and vitamin/minerals) along with bowel and liver cleansing herbs.

BOWEL CLEANSING AND SUPPORT:
Barberry bark (Berberis vulgaris), Cascara sagrada bark (Rhamnus purshiana), Cayenne (Capsicum minimum), Ginger (Zingiber officinale) Golden seal root (Hydrastis canadensis), Lobelia herb and/or seeds (Lobelia inflata), Red raspberry leaves (Rubus idaeus), Turkey rhubarb root (Rheum palmatum), Fennel (Foeniculum vulgari)

LIVER AND GALLBLADDER SUPPORT:

The herbs that compose the liver-gallbladder formula are: barberry, wild yam, cramp bark, fennel seed, ginger, catnip and peppermint.

BLOOD CLEANSING:
Red clover blossoms, chaparral, licorice root, poke root, peach bark, Oregon grape root, stillingia, prickly ash bark, burdock root, and buckthorn bark.

JOINT PAIN:

This usually involves two separate holistic medications:
For joint repair:
Hydrangea root Brigham herb yucca chaparral black walnut, lobelia burdock root, sarsaparilla wild lettuce Valerian wormwood cayenne black cohosh.
For pain and inflammation: Willow tincture.
FOR THE BACTERIAL: INFECTION:
As mentioned earlier in this paper, Cat's Claw is the main "natural antibiotic" used in the battle against the Lyme bacteria. Garlic is also extensively used.

MEDICATION (UNIQUE TO EACH PATIENT BASED ON THE DAMAGE DONE):

For heart damage: Ingredients: Hawthorn berry syrup is made with hawthorn berry juice concentrate using grape brandy and glycerin as aids and preservatives.

For Nerve damage: Ingredients: Black cohosh capsicum hops flowers lobelia skullcap Valerian wood betony mistletoe. I also use one that is used as ear drops: Ingredients: black cohosh blue cohosh blue Vervain skullcap lobelia.

SAUNA, EXERCISE FOR OXYGEN AND HEAT TREATMENTS:
One if the characteristics about the Lyme bacteria is it's intolerance for heat and oxygen. It is now an accepted protocol for Lyme patients to exercise each week, starting at about an a week and building up. This is meant to be strenuous aerobic exercises causing the patients body heat to increase as well as their oxygen load. Most patients report a small Herx response right after the session. For those not able to exercise effectively, a sauna has been found to work well.

Sauna therapy. The Lyme spirochete appears to be very heat sensitive. This is a fact we use to our advantage with near infrared light sauna therapy. It works beautifully with many cases of Lyme disease, and is inexpensive and completely non-toxic. I recommend at least two lamp sauna sessions daily, and they should be 45 to 60 minutes long at 120 degrees F.

FURTHER MEDICATION FOR PAIN:

A combination of Cramp bark and Valerian is used in tincture form as a very powerful and effective muscle relaxer and pain killer. Willow is a very good choice for minor pain and as an anti-inflammatory. CBD in the form of capsules, oils and salves works wonderfully as a quick and efficient pain killer. But again, the best pain killer is finding a cure for the disease.

STRESS MANAGEMENT:

Many different studies lend insight to the role of stress on patients with chronic illness. It is observed that stress also may affect the progression of infection and infectious disease. Research findings have continuously demonstrated a significant role that stress has in bacterial, viral and fungal infection, leading one to conclude that stress is a significant factor in susceptibility, severity, and progression of disease and illness. A growing body of evidence indicates that stress can make arthritis pain worst by increasing sensitivity to pain, reducing coping efforts, and possibly affecting the process of inflammation itself, these direct effects occur through neuroendocrine responses to stress. Stress plays a huge role in chronic illness. Stress is defined as the physical or mental response to demands from the environment, the events that led up to these demands, or the individual's perception of these demands.
If the need is great enough I will recommend talk therapy to give the patient an avenue in dealing with the serious internal issues. I will also discuss various coping mechanisms such as exercise, walking on the forest (also called Forest Bathing by the Japanese), finding hobbies they have not done in years, building a circle of close friends and support groups, both local and online.

LABS FOR MONITORING PROGRESS OF TREATMENT:

As mentioned earlier in this book, the two primary blood test I use for diagnosing and monitoring the progression of the treatment is the Western Blood Serum test and the CD57. Many doctors not trained in Lyme will often opt for the Western Blot Reflex test. This is a very significant mistake as it's success rate for detecting the Lyme bacteria is very poor. Lyme trained doctors will avoid this test and opt for the Serum version.

2.3   Case Histories

CASE HISTORY #1
Heather – Lyme Disease
One of the joys we get at the clinic is the opportunity to be one of the only Lyme-literate clinics in Northern California. It is a sad state to find how little is known about this disease and how poorly the CDC encourages information. It is terribly under reported due to the CDC requirements being absurdly high for what can be classified as Lyme disease.

Fortunately we have Dr. Christopher's knowledge and that of Dr. Burascano, the worlds leading authority on Lyme Disease. He is also very open to alternative medicine as an option for treatment. He has treated over 11,000 patients worldwide. Heather is a common example of a patient with Lyme Disease. Rarely does the patient receive treatment shortly after being bitten by the deer tick as this creature is quite small and most patients will not even realize they have been bitten. In only 20% of the cases does the classic "target" rash show up. In her case she was not diagnosed until about nine years after he initial infection. This results in what we classify as chronic or late term Lyme Disease with secondary infections. This usually results in chronic joint and muscle pain, fatigue, a suppressed immune system along with a variety of other symptoms.

She had been constantly misdiagnosed and was usually labeled with Chronic Fatigue Syndrome, a blanket diagnosis meaning they have no idea what is happening to the patient.

In her case we finally received a blood test back called the Western Blot Test. It showed the bacteria markers for the Lyme Disease organism. We began treatment immediately. One of the most important things to do for chronic Lyme Disease is to deal with the long term damage which is usually with the nerves. We also have to be careful treating the disorder too aggressively as a large die-off of the bacteria can actually harm the patient. We started with the three day cleanse using carrot juice and afterwards she adopted the mucousless diet. The cleansing formulas Lower Bowel and Liver and Gallbladder along with the Kidney formula were also utilized.

45

To aid in the nerve and joint damage we also added the formulas MindTrac, Relax-Eze, St. John's Wort, Complete Tissue and Bone and the Joint formula. To aid in the compromised immune system we added the Adrenal Formula with Immucalm. Within the first month on the program she noticed an increased energy and a lessening of the joint and muscle pain. Her physician in her area has asked for us to consult with him so he can better treat his other patients with this issue. While this program usually takes about a year to complete she continues to improve to this day.

CASE HISTORY #2:

Lara

The patient is a 33 year female who originally came to the clinic presenting a diagnosis of multiple sclerosis. I accepted the previous doctor's assessment and began treating her for this condition. Over the period of a year she saw significant improvement gaining the ability to move out on her own for the first and to hold down a job. Within three weeks of treatment she was no longer using her cane. Since she was doing so well we discontinued the monthly visits and asked her to watch her diet, which was vegan, and to let us know how she was doing. About a year later we saw her again and her old symptoms were returning. I asked if she would be willing to take a series of Lyme blood test and she agreed. The results came back positive. She had been misdiagnosed all along.

We began the outlined Lyme protocol and within weeks she was noticing significant improvement and her CD57 blood test continues to rise.
By 07/18/2018 the CD57 increased to 105 from a previous value of 72 back in April.

CASE HISTORY #3:

Marci

This patient was a 45 year old woman presenting advanced chronic Lyme disease. Symptoms were burning skin, extensive joint and muscle pain, gut issues, weak muscles and systemic candida.

The first protocol involved our 18 day candida cleanse which at the end the patient already noted some improvement in the joint pain. She remained vegan at this point and began the protocol of holistic medication mentioned in this paper along with weekly exercise and saunas. Her energy continued to improve as well a her anxiety and depression disappeared.

She experienced extensive Herxx reactions when I started her later n the Cat's Claw but in time this has significantly disappeared as I increased the dosages. Her latest Western blot showed only one marker remaining. Her last CD57 had risen to a 105 which indicated her immune was starting to fight back successfully.

CASE HISTORY #4:

Donna

This patient was a 53 year old woman who originally presented a very serious case of vaginitis. I ran an STD test and it came back as HSV type 1. She also presented a suppressed immune system, allergies, systemic candida, and painful joints.

She went through the 18 day candida protocol and noticed a slight improvement in her energy and joints. I then proceeded to treat the HSV 1 rash vaginally with immune supporting herbs and St. John's Wort, both internally and topically.

The rash improved but it was a very slow process.
She mentioned an issue with a tick bit in her past so I arraigned for a complete Lyme blood test. The Western Blot Serum showed two bands and the CD57 was a 21, an extremely low value and highly indicative of chronic Lyme.

We started the full Lyme program and in six months her CD57 climbed to a 67, indicating her immune system was beginning to rally. Her vaginitis completely vanished along with a significant improvement in her energy and no longer had any joint pain.

CHAPTER 3

Complimentary results compared with conventional

Conventional: Post-Treatment Lyme Disease Syndrome (PTLDS) represents a subset of patients who remain significantly ill following standard antibiotic therapy for Lyme disease. PTLDS is characterized by a constellation of symptoms that includes severe fatigue, musculoskeletal pain, sleep disturbance, depression, and cognitive problems such as difficulty with short-term memory, speed of thinking, or multi-tasking. In the absence of a direct diagnostic biomarker, PTLDS has been difficult to diagnose by physicians, and its existence has been controversial. However, our clinical research shows that meticulous patient evaluation when used alongside appropriate diagnostic testing can reliably identify patients with typical symptom patterns of PTLDS. Our research also indicates that PTLDS symptoms can significantly impair daily functioning and quality of life. Increased severity of initial illness, the presence of neurologic symptoms, and initial misdiagnosis increase the risk of Post-Treatment Lyme Disease Syndrome. PTLDS is especially common in people that have had neurologic involvement. The rates of Post-Treatment Lyme Disease Syndrome after neurologic involvement may be as high as 20% or even higher. Without neurologic symptoms, the rates of Post-Treatment Lyme Disease Syndrome tend to be in the 10% to 20% range.

Complementary: Holistic treatment should entail well-selected remedies, including clinical chosen for the patient, intercurrent miasmatic remedies and acute remedies for side effects and die-off symptoms. These remedies should be changed according to the patient's responses. Then once 75% of the symptoms are taken care of and the patients can manage the acute flair ups (which should lessen in frequency after time as their health is restored) the Lyme disease is eradicated and their health is restored. At that point constitutional remedies should be prescribed at least once a year to maintain the patient's health.

In each of my patients who followed the program as prescribed, we saw 100% success with eradication of the symptoms as well as any sign clinically of the bacteria's presence.

References – Misdiagnosis of Lyme disease

1. Goldenberg DL. Fibromyalgia, chronic fatigue syndrome, and myofascial pain syndrome. Curr Opin Rheumatol, 6(2), 223-233 (1994).

2. Clauw DJ, Chrousos GP. Chronic pain and fatigue syndromes: overlapping clinical and neuroendocrine features and potential pathogenic mechanisms. Neuroimmunomodulation, 4(3), 134-153 (1997).

3. Naesens R, Vermeiren S, Van Schaeren J, Jeurissen A. False positive Lyme serology due to syphilis: report of 6 cases and review of the literature. Acta Clin Belg, 66(1), 58-59 (2011).

4. Cimmino MA, Salvarani C. Polymyalgia rheumatica and giant cell arteritis. Baillieres Clin Rheumatol, 9(3), 515-527 (1995).

5. Paparone PW. Polymyalgia rheumatica or Lyme disease? How to avoid misdiagnosis in older patients. Postgrad Med, 97(1), 161-164, 167-170 (1995).

6. Schwartzberg M, Weber CA, Musico J. Lyme borreliosis presenting as a polymyalgia rheumatica-like syndrome. Br J Rheumatol, 34(4), 392-393 (1995).

7. Daoud KF, Barkhuizen A. Rheumatic mimics and selected triggers of fibromyalgia. Curr Pain Headache Rep, 6(4), 284-288 (2002).

8. Steere AC, Malawista SE, Snydman DR et al. Lyme arthritis: an epidemic of oligoarticular arthritis in children and adults in three connecticut communities. Arthritis Rheum, 20(1), 7-17 (1977).

9. Feder HM, Jr., Whitaker DL. Misdiagnosis of erythema migrans. Am J Med, 99(4), 412-419 (1995).

10. Nowakowski J, McKenna D, Nadelman RB et al. Failure of treatment with cephalexin for Lyme disease. Arch Fam Med, 9(6), 563-567 (2000).

11. Plotkin SA. Correcting a public health fiasco: The need for a new vaccine against Lyme disease. Clinical infectious diseases : an official publication of the Infectious Diseases Society of America, 52 Suppl 3, s271-275 (2011).

12.Brinar VV, Habek M. Rare infections mimicking MS. Clin Neurol Neurosurg, (2010).

13.Calabresi PA. Diagnosis and management of multiple sclerosis. Am Fam Physician, 70(10), 1935-1944 (2004).

14.Trojano M, Paolicelli D. The differential diagnosis of multiple sclerosis: classification and clinical features of relapsing and progressive neurological syndromes. Neurol Sci, 22 Suppl 2, S98-102 (2001).

15.Fallon BA, Keilp JG, Corbera KM et al. A randomized, placebo-controlled trial of repeated IV antibiotic therapy for Lyme encephalopathy. Neurology, 70(13), 992-1003 (2008).

16.Paparone PW. Polymyalgia rheumatica or Lyme disease? How to avoid misdiagnosis in older patients. Postgrad Med, 97(1), 161-164, 167-170 (1995).

17.Schwartzberg M, Weber CA, Musico J. Lyme borreliosis presenting as a polymyalgia rheumatica-like syndrome. Br J Rheumatol, 34(4), 392-393 (1995).

18.Jennings F, Lambert E, Fredericson M. Rheumatic diseases presenting as sports-related injuries. Sports Med, 38(11), 917-930 (2008).

19.Cameron DJ. Consequences of treatment delay in Lyme disease. J Eval Clin Pract, 13(3), 470-472 (2007).

Hu LT. Lyme Disease. Ann Intern Med. 2016 Nov 1;165(9):677.

• Kowalski TJ, Tata S, Berth W, Mathiason MA, Agger WA Antibiotic treatment duration and long-term outcomes of patients with early Lyme disease from a Lyme disease-hyperendemic area. Clin Infect Dis. 2010;50(4):512-520.

• Sanchez E, Vannier E, Wormser GP, Hu LT. Diagnosis, treatment, and prevention of Lyme disease, human granulocytic anaplasmosis, and babesiosis: A review.JAMA. 2016 Apr 26;315(16):1767-77.

• Stupica D, Lusa L, Ruzić-Sabljić E, Cerar T, Strle F. Treatment of erythema migrans with doxycycline for 10 days versus 15 days. Clin Infect Dis. 2012;55(3):343-350.

About The Author

Dr. Earendil M. Spindelilus D.N.M., M.H., C.R. - Traditional Naturopath, Holistic Practitioner, Clinical Master Herbalist, Certified Nutritionist, Certified Reflexology, Member of Plant Savers of America, Member of American Botanical Council.

I hold a Doctorate degree in Natural Medicine. I have also been a lecturer since 1999. Board Certified Diplomate of Natural Medicine. Member of the American Council of Holistic Medicine.

I have always had a deep and abiding interest in the Plant Kingdom. Even very young I loved the way the herbs held the mystery of healing within them and how I could learn about them. I traveled around the world learning from different cultures their own unique floras and how they incorporated them into their daily lives. With each new herb I learned how special the world is and how Nature supplies us with all we need. In the 1990s I decided to take my education further and enrolled in the School and Natural Healing, the College of Herbal Medicine. I graduated in 1999 with my Master Herbalist. I have also studied with the New Eden School of Natural Medicine where I completed my Doctorate in Natural Medicine. To date, my wife and I have run two medical centers for natural healing. It has always been a great joy meeting with our patients. We are all meant to live a happy, healthy life and when we allow our body to perform it's innate ability to heal itself then this can happen. I am also a past board member of the Reflexology Association of California as well as a published author/writer of numerous holistic books and articles. I am also a past host of a holistic radio show.

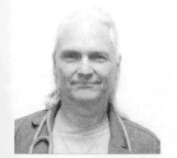

Made in United States
North Haven, CT
25 July 2023

39503770R00039